Patiently Waiting

Patiently Waiting

Diane Heupel

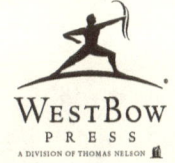

WestBow
P R E S S
A DIVISION OF THOMAS NELSON

WestBow Press books may be ordered through booksellers or by contacting:

WestBow Press
A Division of Thomas Nelson
1663 Liberty Drive
Bloomington, IN 47403
www.westbowpress.com
1-(866) 928-1240

Because of the dynamic nature of the Internet, any web addresses or
links contained in this book may have changed since publication and
may no longer be valid. The views expressed in this work are solely those
of the author and do not necessarily reflect the views of the publisher,
and the publisher hereby disclaims any responsibility for them.

Any people depicted in stock imagery provided by Thinkstock are models,
and such images are being used for illustrative purposes only.

Certain stock imagery © Thinkstock.

ISBN: 978-1-4497-4791-6 (sc)

Library of Congress Control Number: 2012907935

Printed in the United States of America

WestBow Press rev. date: 5/9/2012

Dear Reader:

The reason I wrote this book, I am hoping the experience that I went through, which wasn't easy, that it would help some moms out there that have had trouble bearing a child. It wasn't easy to go through what I did, but I was determined and didn't give up. It was with the help of the Lord that we were able to finally have a baby, which was truly a miracle from the Lord.

If any Mom ever wants to talk to me about what I went through, I would be willing to visit with her and try to help her out the best way that I could.

Through my experience, I believe the Lord has made me more compassionate toward other people.

This book is dedicated to Elmer's family, Diane's family, our dear relatives and friends, and especially to mothers who have miscarried.

Elmer and I were married June 29, 1974 at Our Redeemer's Lutheran Church in Williston, North Dakota. We were so much in love and thought we had the world by the tail. Much to our surprise we didn't have the world by the tail. We had many ups and downs.

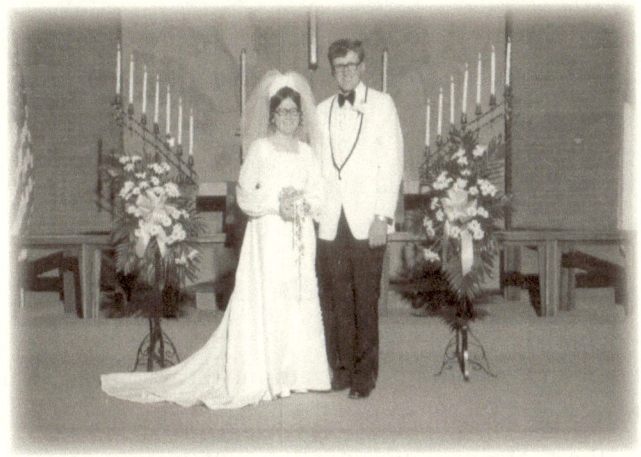

We both accepted the Lord as our Savior in September of 1976. I know now that without the Lord we would never have made it through all our trials.

We decided to wait on having a family until we got somewhat established in farming. When we did decide to try and have a baby, it took some time to become pregnant. I finally got pregnant when I was 34 years old. I started spotting one day so Elmer took me to one of the nearest clinics and the doctor confirmed my pregnancy. This appointment was on December 22, 1982. That was such a beautiful Christmas present for both of us. My father-in-law cried when Elmer told him, as he was so happy for us.

The local doctor would not take care of pregnant moms so he referred me to a doctor in Bismarck.

I made a doctor's appointment for January of 1983 with an obstetrician-gynecologist for a physical. I went to a lady doctor for a very thorough exam and she reconfirmed my pregnancy. She said everything looked fine except for the heartbeat. She had me come to the hospital in February as an outpatient for an ultrasound to find the heartbeat. Ultrasound was really neat. I could see our baby moving around. The baby was very active. The doctor also decided to do an amniocentesis test because of our age. The test took three weeks to come back. When it did come back, the doctor called and talked to Elmer. She told him the good news. Everything was fine and we were going to become parents of a baby girl on August 16, 1983.

I went back for my pre-natal checkup on March 18, 1983. The doctor gave me a good report. I was gaining just the right amount of weight and also the baby's heartbeat was very strong. We got back to our farm that evening and I went to the bathroom. I was spotting and when I saw that I was terrified. I called the doctor and she sent me to bed. The next morning I was passing chunks. She said I could get up on Monday, but not to overdo it. Monday and Tuesday I didn't feel that great.

Tuesday evening Elmer had a meeting at Elgin, ND. I asked him if I could ride along as something kept telling me not to stay home alone. So I went to visit his folks while he was at the meeting. I was there about an hour when I was going to get up and go to the bathroom.

I just screamed, "My water broke!" "Mom, call Elmer." Mom got so nervous she called the wrong number first. She finally got Elmer and he came right away. Then she called the doctor and the doctor said we should come to the Emergency Room entrance. Mom gave me a blanket as I was saturated. It was a long 77 miles to the hospital in Bismarck, ND. Then Elmer got nervous and missed the turn so it took longer to get to the hospital. We finally got there.

A nurse was waiting there with a wheelchair at the door. I was fine until I saw her then I started to cry. I said, "Am I going to lose my baby?" She said, "Don't worry, dear, they will take care of you." It made me upset as she didn't answer my question.

They took me to a room. The doctor came to the hospital right away. They found the baby's heartbeat, but it wasn't as strong as the Friday before. The doctor was honest with us. She didn't give us much hope. I tried to sleep that night, but couldn't—all I could do was cry.

Elmer stayed at a motel that night and came up the next morning. The doctor came in and asked how I was doing. "I said I'm doing fine. I'm going home with Elmer today." "Oh, no you are not, you will have to have strict bed rest today."

The doctor sent me to ultrasound as she said if I didn't lose that much of my amniotic fluid I would have to spend the rest of my pregnancy in bed. I was in my 19th week so that meant 21 weeks flat on my back. Elmer decided one week my folks would have to come and help and the next week his folks. The parents would have to keep taking turns.

Elmer went down with me to ultrasound. Elmer and I saw our daughter was still moving, but not like before. They said I had lost too much amniotic fluid. They said I had to go back to my room and lay flat on my back. The doctor figured there was still a chance, but she wanted to watch me in case an infection set in.

Elmer decided to leave for home. We cried so hard before he left. I couldn't take it, so I knew our Pastor from Church was working at the State Capitol, so I called him and told him what was happening. He was in my hospital room within a half an hour praying with me and giving me spiritual support.

I was so concerned about Elmer, too, so we prayed he would have a safe trip home.

In the afternoon I called my aunt who lived in town. She came up to be with me. My aunt said it wasn't fair I was losing my baby. I was across the hall from a lady who had twin girls. My aunt said she should go and ask her if I could please have one of the twin girls.

I drank so much water that day I was in the hospital. I always had said if I ever go to a hospital, I never want to use a bed pan. Well, guess what I had to keep calling the nurse all day. A bed pan!! What fun!! Around 5:00 p.m. my temperature started rising. I was getting an infection. I called Pastor and told him when he went back to Elgin that he should get a hold of Elmer and tell him. I cried some more. I've never cried for such a long period of time.

Around 9:30 p.m. a nurse came in to find the heartbeat. She worked for a long time. I couldn't hear anything. She didn't say anything about it to me. She just sat by my bedside and visited with me for a long time. I slept a little better that night. The next morning about 6:30 a.m. I woke up with pain. It started coming every few mintues apart. I called the nurse at 7:00 a.m. and told her.

Even though I was in pain I was so hungry. I called for breakfast, and they said it would be coming. They just didn't bring it so I got hungrier and ate the orange I had left over from the night before.

Then the nurses came in and moved me next to the nurse's station so they could watch me closer. I asked the head nurse if I could have my aunt come up and be with me.

She said, "sure." So I called my aunt. I called Elmer and told him I was sure I was in labor. Then the nurse came in and asked me if I minded if a male nurse that was in student nursing could come in to take care of me during labor. I hesitated at first, but then I thought they have to learn, too. I found out later I was glad the Lord had sent him to take care of me. He was so sympathetic and understanding about my situation. So I had him on one side of the bed and my aunt on the other side of the bed. The pains were coming stronger and I was getting sicker. I was freezing cold. I kept asking for another blanket. I had 6 blankets on me and I was still cold so the male nurse said he would get the 7th blanket for me. The nurse warmed up the blanket in the microwave oven. Then I finally warmed up. He helped me with my breathing, but then my arms and legs started going numb. Then I started sweating. Then Aunt Norma spooned ice into my mouth and put a wet washrag on my forehead. Then I felt sicker. I said "Hurry, I'm going to throw up," and I did, too. I found out that is why they didn't bring me breakfast. I wasn't suppose to eat after I had gone into labor.

My aunt kept saying, "Diane, why do you have to suffer so?" The male nurse said he could share my hurts as he just went through some real hurts. He was engaged to a girl and she wanted to get married right away, but he wanted to wait and finish school first. She wouldn't wait for him, so they broke up and he hadn't gotten over this yet so in a sense we shared our problems with one another. He could tell the way I talked that Elmer and I were very close to one another. Labor was getting more intense. The pain was excruciating. The RN came in and said it wouldn't be long. I was dilated to 10 and they would call the doctor. The doctor came up to my room in 10 minutes. I delivered around noon on March 24, 1983. The doctor asked me if I wanted to see the baby and I chose not to, but she didn't encourage me to see the baby either. To this day, I wish I would have held my daughter and had a memorial service for her.

The doctor said our baby was dead and I had just delivered a baby girl. So she took off running to the Lab with everything.

Diane Heupel

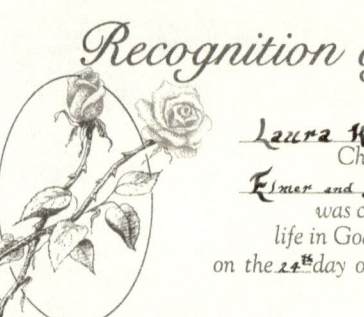

Recognition of Life

Laura Kay Heupel
Child of
Elmer and Diane Heupel
was called to
life in God's Kingdom
on the 24th day of march 19 83

Before I formed you in the womb,
I knew you.
Before you came to birth
I consecrated you.

Jeremiah 1:5

They finally brought me dinner and I barely got to finish and they needed my bed. So Aunt Norma helped me move from 2nd floor to 4th floor.

One of my Christian friends came in and hugged me and then all I could do was cry some more. My friend stayed with me until Elmer came and then we cried some more.

A social worker came to see me while I was in the hospital every day. She had me tell her what was bothering me which really helped.

That afternoon I had fallen asleep for awhile and when I woke up, Pastor and his wife were standing by my bedside. They had driven 77 miles just to see me and pray with me and give me some spiritual support. Pastor told me they knew how I felt as they had lost twin boys. He started to cry with me. That really helped me, to know that someone could know and share the same kind of loss with me.

My girlfriend, her husband and son came to visit with Elmer and I in the evening and brought us some flowers. They were good friends of mine. They were just ready to leave and here came two couples from our Church at Elgin to be with us. They brought us a beautiful plant. That really touched our hearts they drove all that way to spend some time with us.

Several friends and relatives called that evening to extend their sympathy. Elmer spent the evening with my aunt and uncle.

The next morning the doctor came to see both of us. She told us both she was sorry and she cried with us. She said Elmer had to see a social worker before we left the hospital. She wanted both of us going home not feeling like it was something we had done to cause the loss of our baby. The social worker told us there was a group in Bismarck called Compassionate Friends (a support group) for couples who have lost babies where we could go for further help.

Now it was time for my release from the hospital. I had to go home with empty arms. I was going to get dressed and my slacks were missing. How could I leave the hospital with no slacks? When Elmer brought my clothes, the slacks weren't on the hanger, just my top. So we decided we had to call my aunt to see if I could borrow a pair of her slacks. When I called all I could do was laugh. I couldn't tell her what I needed because I was laughing so hard. Elmer had to take the phone and tell her what I needed. At least I could laugh again. Elmer had to go back up to my aunt and uncle's house and get me a pair of slacks to wear.

Now it was time to leave the hospital. I had to say goodbye to the male nurse and give him some homemade buns from my aunt. I think the nurse that was taking me out in the wheelchair was upset with me because I wanted to go and see him. Elmer drove up to the front door to get me. Then we had to go to Hoskins Meyer Floral Shop and pick up a bouquet from my sister and her family. It was just beautiful. Then we were on our way back to our farm south of New Leipzig without our baby daughter which we named Laura Kay Heupel. She weighed only 8 oz.

When we got to Elgin we stopped at Mom and Dad Heupel's. We had dinner with them. And, of course, we cried. Elmer asked his Mom where his sister was that day. She usually came to eat with the folks as she worked at the local bank. Mom said, "She has a doctor's appointment. She thinks she is pregnant again." Boy, wow that hurt. Here we had just come home from the hospital without our baby and his sister is going to have another baby. "Why," I ask, but I get no answers.

After dinner we went home. On our dining room table was this beautiful Easter lily. Elmer had bought it for me. We just took each other in our arms and cried and cried.

Shortly after we came home, Mom and Dad Larsen came to help. They lived at Epping, ND. They drove 235 miles to our farm. We cried some more after my parents came. So many people called that day. Dad Larsen finally took the phone away from me as I was getting so weak and pale looking. The folks did the cooking and the cleaning. We had 16 calls and 17 visitors. Mom and Dad Larsen couldn't believe how caring and loving all of our friends were.

I couldn't go down our basement steps to take a shower, so Dad Larsen drove me 13 miles every other day to Elmer's folks at Elgin so I could take a shower. It felt so good to get out of the house and get some fresh air.

One day Dad Larsen was going to take a nap in the one bedroom upstairs. He came down and said he couldn't sleep. I said, "Why?" Dad said, "Because the baby's bathtub was laying on the bed upstairs." That is the only thing we had for the baby and we had gotten it from Elmer's sister to use.

A week after my miscarriage I had to go back for a checkup. I just cried when I saw the nurse. She said, "I'm sorry. I know how you feel as I lost a baby, too." That seemed to help. She gave me some information to read on miscarriages. It explained it quite well as several people asked if we were going to have a Memorial Service for our daughter. We didn't know what to do, but the papers the nurse gave me said that you don't. To this day we regret that we didn't have a memorial service. We just should of went ahead and did what we felt like doing.

The doctor came in and checked me and I cried some more. She said I was doing fine and there was really no reason why I had miscarried. She read the lab report to me. The baby appeared to be normal and healthy and every organ in her body was formed.

So we had no answers—all we knew was that Laura was up in Heaven and Jesus is taking care of her. We never got to see her except on ultrasound. We never got to hold her, but we love her very much and we are waiting to see her in heaven some day. Many people gave us cards and readings that helped ease our sorrow. Some of these were:

"I will lift up mine eyes unto the hills, from whence cometh my help."

Psalm 121:1

"The Lord is nigh unto them that are of a broken heart."

Psalm 34:18

A BABY'S SECRET

I am just a little feller, Who didn't quite make it there.

I went straight to be with Jesus, But I'm waiting for you there.

Don't you fret about me mommy, I'm of all God's lambs most blest.

I'd have loved to stay there with you; But the Shepherd knows what's best..By J.C. Brumfield

One verse I kept repeating that really helps is Phillipians 4:13.

"I can do all things through Christ which strengthens me."

So many women told me they had miscarried. I had known some of these ladies for a long time. That seemed to be a comfort to us to know someone else had gone through the same trials as we were going through.

One of the hardest things for me to do was to go back to church. But I knew I had to go to church again. I guess I knew when I saw my friends I would cry. They came and grabbed me and hugged me and it made me feel so good, but of course I cried which helped me through my grief. It helps to get it out and not keep everything inside of you. But yet there were friends that wouldn't say anything to us. It not only happened at church, but it happened everywhere we went. I guess they were scared and didn't know what to say. I've learned if you don't know what to say just go over to that person that is hurting and give them a hug and hold them in your arms and cry with them.

We were told that we had to wait six months before we tried to have another baby. Elmer still felt the doctor should have checked into our situation further and did some testing to find out what really caused the miscarriage. We were determined to try again.

In the Spring of 1984 I conceived for the second time. This time I went to Hettinger to the doctor. I was spotting every so often. I was told my baby was due in February of 1985.

In June of 1984 another gal and I went to Hettinger to attend a Share Support Group. This group was for families that lost babies. It was very informative and a comfort to share with one another.

I had a complete physical in August of 1984 and the doctor confirmed my pregnancy. But they couldn't find the heartbeat again. So off to ultrasound I went. They did find the heart beat on ultrasound and he said everything looked fine. I went back again in September for a monthly checkup. The doctor gave me a good report. Later in September I developed a bladder infection so I had to go and see the doctor. I was put on antibiotics.

Everything was going fine until October 7, 1984. I got up to go to church and to finish my dinner preparations. We were going to have company after church. I kept getting this pain every so often, but I tried to put it out of my mind. I went to church and I asked my girlfriend what she thought. She said she thought I should call my doctor. I called the doctor and he said I should go home and put my feet up. He thought I had what is called Braxton Hicks. It happens when your uterus enlarges.

We had Mission Fest at our church and we had invited the missionaries through Steer, Inc. to join us for dinner. Elmer went to find the missionaries and told them to come out for dinner anyway as I had everything ready. So Elmer and I went home and I sat in the recliner and put my feet up. The missionaries came out after church were with Campus Crusade for Christ.

The lady missionary had been a doctor in the Philippines. She said that I might be lacking progesterone. So we visited while we ate. Elmer brought me my food to the recliner. All of a sudden I got an excruciating pain and I went to the bathroom. I lost all my water again. I told our company I was sorry, but we would have to leave for the hospital. The missionaries prayed with us and we left. We didn't even get to eat our dessert.

I kept telling Elmer to drive faster as I was in so much pain. Half ways to Hettinger I remembered my pie for our dessert was still in the oven on warm.

We got to Hettinger to the Emergency Room, another doctor was on call. They got me ready for bed and put an IV on me right away. They couldn't find the heartbeat. Then my doctor came to the hospital. He said that I was dilated to 10 and it wouldn't be long before I would deliver. Then I asked him if I could be lacking progesterone. The doctor left and kept calling and checking on me.

I spent the night in the Hettinger Hospital. Elmer stayed with me until about 5:30 p.m. that evening. The doctor called the hospital at 12:30 a.m., but nothing had happened. Of course I did my share of crying again.

The next morning they checked me and were thinking about doing a D & C. But after he checked me, he decided to induce labor. They still couldn't find a heartbeat.

Boy, I thought I was going to die. I never had so much pain. The doctor left for New England to see patients that day at 9:00 a.m. He thought it wouldn't be long before I delivered my baby. In the morning I was laying in such pain and the nurse came in and asked if I wanted company. I said, "Sure!" Here it was my Aunt. Then we started to cry.

My Aunt and Uncle from Bismarck had stopped at our farm. They wanted to see me and Elmer told them he had to take me to Hettinger the day before to the hospital as I was losing our second baby. So my aunt and uncle decided they would drive to Hettinger to see me. This would be the second time my aunt would be with me when I was losing a baby.

Elmer was at home working on the quonset door when my relatives stopped by. We had had a lot of damage in a storm that had gone through our farmyard in August.

I was glad my relatives came all the way to Hettinger to see me. About 1:00 p.m. Elmer came. Nothing had happened. I told him to rub my back as I had such back pain.

At 3:00 p.m. the nurse said that she was leaving. I didn't want her to go off duty as she had been so nice to me. A new nurse came on duty and she wouldn't let me get up, so back to the good old bed pan again.

The doctor came back from New England at 5:00 p.m. He could not believe I had not had the baby yet. He told Elmer he would have to leave the room. The doctor decided he had to pull the baby. That hurt so bad. Elmer heard me screaming as he was standing out in the hallway.

I had a baby boy. He weighed 10 oz. I just started crying so hard. Elmer came back in and we just held each other and started crying so hard together.

The doctor took our baby son to the Lab and he said that he would send him into the State Lab for an autopsy. We did not see our son and we were not given the option to see him.

The doctor felt so sorry for us so he ordered Elmer supper so he could eat with me. Elmer left the Hospital at 9:00 p.m.

We named our son Loren Lee.

Diane Heupel

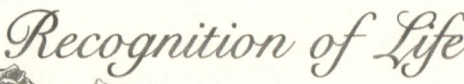

Recognition of Life

<u>Lorin Lee Heupel</u>
Child of
<u>Elmer and Diane Heupel</u>
was called to
life in God's Kingdom
on the <u>8th</u> day of <u>October</u> 19 <u>84</u>

Before I formed you in the womb,
I knew you.
Before you came to birth
I consecrated you.

Jeremiah 1:5

Then I couldn't pass my placenta. They brought me a form to sign about 8:00 p.m. The form was consent to a D & C that I would have performed on me the next morning. I prayed so hard as I didn't want to go through that yet. At 10:30 p.m. the Lord answered my prayer. I went to the bathroom and I was able to pass my placenta. I put on the nurse's light. She came running as she thought I had fainted. I said "No!" I told the nurse that I knew that she was about to call the doctor and I wanted you to tell him that I had passed my placenta.

The next morning I was released from the hospital to go home again with empty arms. Mom Heupel was at the farm to help a couple of days. Then my folks came to help again. I was glad to see Mom and Dad Larsen and was grateful for all the help.

Once again, I went back for a checkup. They could find nothing wrong. The body was fully developed. All the organs were formed. The only thing the doctor could think of that was wrong was that I had Chlamydia infection, which causes you to lose babies. So both Elmer and I were put on antibiotics as one partner can give it to another partner. Elmer and I started reading up on Chlamydia. The more we read on it, we were almost sure we didn't have it.

After I got home from the hospital, I had 24 calls and 5 visitors. I also received several flower bouquets and some food.

Diane Heupel

Here are some poems and writings I received that were in the sympathy cards:

THE WEAVER

My life is but a weaving

Between my Lord and me,

I cannot choose the colors

He worketh steadily............ By B.M. Franklin

ALONG THE ROAD

By Robert Browning Hamilton

FOR ETERNITY

How could one comfort, What words could one say?

That precious, tiny life has slipped away

Back to the loving Father's arms so soon

You'd scarcely know it has been in the room....................

Author Unknown

I had wanted to go home on Monday evening from the hospital, as I was to help with a baby shower. Needless to say, the Doctor wouldn't let me.

Elmer's cousin came out to spend some time with me on Thursday afternoon as Elmer had to go to court with a neighbor who was going through a divorce. That afternoon Dad Heupel was trying to help haul manure in the corral and he got the loader bucket up too high and tore down the electric wires. Thank goodness he didn't get electrocuted.

Mom and Dad Larsen came down to help out again. It was very hard on the Parents and us as we had just gone through losing the second baby.

Some of our friends gave us the name of a specialist in Bismarck. So in January of 1985 we wrote a letter to this specialist about my problems and asked him for a second opinion. In February of 1985 we went to Bismarck for our first appointment. We discussed what previously had happened with the Specialist. He had a Chlamydia culture taken and a vaginal culture taken. Both tests came back negative. In March he scheduled me to go to the hospital as an outpatient for a hysterosalpinogram. The doctor was looking for an abnormal growth in the uterus. He called it a septum. He figured when I would get so big, that would puncture the fluid and then I would lose the baby. I went in for the test. They shoot dye up you for the test and then they take an x-ray. They wouldn't let Elmer in as it was an x-ray. It was a very painful test. I just clenched my teeth. The x-ray said my uterus was normal.

I think the Doctor was stunned. Then he told Elmer and I to go to the clinic for chromosome tests. So we did. They were very expensive. Our insurance wouldn't cover the tests. They were $400 a piece. Those tests came back negative. All together between Elmer and I we had 30 tests.

The next step would be to have a progesterone test run. So in April I went back to the Lab for that test. That test came back that I was very deficient in progesterone. My level was down to 7 and it should have been 20. When I found out I just cried. The Doctor was very shocked when he found out I had low progesterone.

So he had to put me on progesterone to conceive.

On *October 11, 1985* Elmer and I found out we were pregnant with our third child.

On *December 3, 1985* Elmer and I got to listen to the heartbeat.

I felt the first kick on my birthday on *January 22, 1986*.

Elmer felt our baby kicking on *Valentine's Day*. I had to be on progesterone for the first 13 weeks of my pregnancy.

On *March 25, 1986* I went to the hospital for ultrasound. I was so upset with the receptionist at ultrasound as she didn't have the specimen jars. Elmer had to go over to the clinic and get one while I registered. Ultrasound is so neat. You can see your baby moving around. When I was finished they told me I could finally go to the bathroom.

I had to report to the clinic by 1:00 p.m. I saw a different doctor. The doctor said that I was doing okay, but my cervix was getting shorter and I had to go home and be on strict bed rest. I also was supposed to take brethine every six hours to prevent labor from coming on. All I could do was get up to eat, go to the bathroom and take a shower. We didn't like his diagnosis and also he couldn't find the baby's heartbeat with the dopler. So I cried and went home to bed.

On *March 26*th Mom and Dad Heupel came out. Mom made us dinner and supper. Dad helped Elmer outside. It was a long boring day laying around.

On *March 27ᵗʰ* I went back to the Doctor. Here comes a different doctor in again. We said we want to see the doctor I had as my doctor. We wanted to see my doctor as we wanted a second opinion. So my doctor came in and checked my cervix. Unfortunately, the other doctor was right. My doctor said my cervix had thinned out and I was dilated to one. So he gave me brethine for 25 more days.

He said they could not stitch me up as it was too late in my pregnancy and I might get an infection. So before I left the room he made me call my aunt in Bismarck. The doctor said I could not leave Bismarck—I had to stay with my aunt and uncle and be on strict bed rest. When Elmer left me there, all I could do was cry. Elmer could only come down to see me on Sundays as he was busy with calving.

March 28-My cousin was home for Easter vacation. So we had a good visit. Our Pastor called to say they prayed for me in church and to see how I was doing. My friend from Elgin called. We both cried. Mom and Dad Heupel brought my clothes. My friend from Wilton came to visit.

March 29-I laid around. The days get so long. I'm scared and the medicine makes me feel awful. I get so weak and shaky and my heart beats fast. I received one letter and had two phone calls today. That really brightens my day.

March 30-It is Easter Sunday today. My aunt, uncle and cousin went to Church. I listened to Church on the radio.

It is the first Easter Elmer and I have been apart since we were married. Elmer and Mom Larsen called me. My cousin left to go back to Minneapolis. I miss her.

March 31-It is another long day. I did some crafts. I also watched a couple of programs on television. I called one of my friends and I received two cards in the mail.

April 1-I folded towels for my aunt. I did some crafts again. I also read some in a book. I received four cards and letters. I washed my hair and I got one phone call.

April 2-I got two phone calls and one letter. I did some more crafts and did some reading. I watched television. It rained a lot today, so it was a very dreary day.

April 3-I went to the doctor I had lost two pounds. He said to keep taking the awful medicine. My cervix is softening, but I'm still dilated to one. The doctor feels once the contractions start, dilation will go fast. So he gave me orders to stay in Bismarck another week. The baby's heartbeat was 160, which was good. I spotted some from his pelvic exam. I never had done that before. I received two letters. My friend from New Leipzig brought me some things from back home. She also brought me three beautiful carnations. She stayed and had supper with my aunt and I.

April 4-I wrote seven letters today. I also did some crafts and read some. My aunt, Ginger (the dog) and I took a long nap. I received four phone calls. A friend from

New Leipzig and her brother stopped by to see me, they brought me a pink and blue carnation.

April 5-I finished the book that my friend gave me. I got three letters and four phone calls. My sister-in-law, nephew and niece and Mom Heupel came to visit me. I watched television in the evening.

April 6-I didn't feel the best after I got up. My aunt stayed home with me in the morning. She didn't go along with my uncle to Church. Elmer came about noon. It was so good to see him after ten days. I cried so hard when he left again. I wanted to go home so bad.

April 7-I worked on crafts most of the day. So the time went fast today. Mom and Dad Larsen called me in the evening.

April 8-I worked on crafts today.

There was a major snowstorm the week of *April 13th*. I was blocked in at my aunt and uncle's.

On *April 17th* after my aunt and I ate supper, I went to the bathroom and I was spotting. My aunt took me to the hospital right away. They tried to stop the labor, but couldn't get it stopped. I had to have the neighbors find Elmer so he could come down. Elmer stayed with me in my room on Thursday night.

Friday morning, *April 18th* at 7:50 a.m. CST, Krista Marie was born. She weighed 4 lbs. 10 oz. and was 18 ½ inches long. The nurses took her right away to put her in an incubator. I was so scared to go and see her as I thought she would be hooked up to all kinds of tubes. It wasn't as bad as I thought. Krista was hooked up to oxygen. We could only stick our finger through a side hole in the incubator and hold her fingers and talk to her.

Diane Heupel

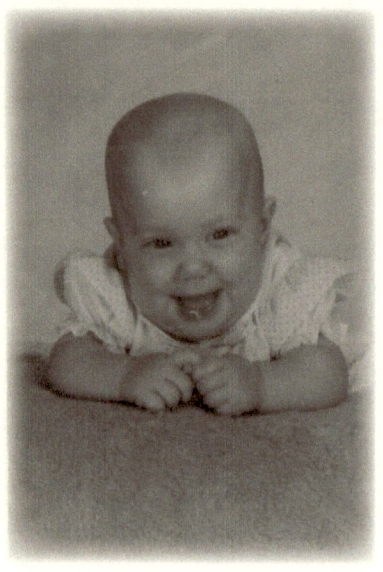

The doctor thought our baby would only weigh three pounds, but Krista fooled him. She weighed over four pounds. He also said she was a couple of months premature, but the ICU doctor thought she was only a month premature.

April 20-Krista's blood sugar was up and down. They put an IV in her head to maintain her weight. Her billirubin count was 11.6 so they started a light. Her urine output picked up and she had a good sign on her breathing.

April 21-Krista was doing very well. They took the IV in her belly button out. This was to register her blood gases. They also took her off oxygen today.

April 22-I had to start feeding her water. I could just give her less than an ounce every three hours. She was sucking very good. Her billirubin count was up to 12.9.

April 23-Her billy lights were still on. She drank one ounce of milk today.

April 24- I got to start nursing Krista today.

April 25-Krista was taken out of the incubator and put in a crib.

April 29-Krista's weight went down to four lbs. 3 ¼ ounces. My milk was starting to let up. I went to a bath demonstration for babies. I got to take Krista along.

April 30-Today I had to start using the breast shield. Krista nursed 15 cc in the evening.

May 1-Krista's weight was back up to 4 lbs. 5 oz. She nursed 10 cc in the morning and 5 cc in the afternoon. I gave Krista her first bath. I could walk her down the hall now.

May 3-Krista slept through the night really good. She is gaining weight.

May 4-Krista is nursing 45 cc every three hours. She has good pink color. She weighs 4 lbs. 7 oz. and she is sleeping really well.

May 5-Krista weighs 4 lbs. 8 oz.

May 9-We brought Krista home. She weighs 4 lbs. 12 oz. She slept all the way home.

When Elmer or I or close relatives went into see Krista in ICU, we had to scrub up before we went in to see her and we also had to put on gowns.

When my aunt came up with me one day, Krista heard my aunt's talking and Krista turned her head. My aunt could not believe how strong she was, yet so little.

One nurse that worked at the Hospital and that was a good friend of ours, stopped by to see Krista every day. She was shocked the day she came up and she couldn't find Krista in the incubator. She couldn't believe that they had moved her to the crib already. It was nice to see my good friend every day. Every once in awhile we would go down to the cafeteria for lunch.

Krista was so little that she fit in her dad's palm of his hand.

When Krista was in the hospital we got several phone calls. We also had a lot of visitors. A lot of the visitors were from our church.

Once we got Krista home, she really started to grow. When I took Krista back to the doctor for her first weight check, the nurse weighed her. The doctor thought the nurse had weighed her wrong. So he went and weighed her again. He couldn't believe it, that on May 16th she weighed 5 lbs. 5 ½ oz and she was 19 ½ inches long.

The neighbors were waiting for us to come home. One neighbor went upstairs in her house to look out to see if our car was home.

Some of the comments when we got Krista home were that she was so little and she was so cute. Her dad couldn't believe all the hair that she had.

May 30th I took Krista back for another weight check. She weighed 7 lbs. 1 ¼ oz. and was 21 inches long.

Krista started looking at books when she was one month old

At two months old, Krista started smiling at her Mom and Dad.

When Krista turned three months old, she started sleeping all night.

Several ladies had a baby shower for us at our Church in June. Krista received a lot of nice baby gifts.

We had Krista dedicated to the Lord in July of 1986.

On *July 11th*, I took Krista back for another weight check. She weighed 10 lbs. 14 oz. and was 21 inches long.

Krista found that she had two hands when she turned four months old. On September 1, 1986 Krista started holding up her head and she also picked up her first toy, which was a little pink rabbit.

On *September 27, 1986* Krista got to go to her first wedding in Lemmon, South Dakota.

On *October 3, 1986* our girl started laughing.

On October 5th, Krista got to go to her first auction sale. She enjoyed looking out the windows of the car when we were driving and looking at the cows and the trees.

The fall of 1986 we took Krista on her first trip. We went to see her aunt, uncle and cousins in Algona, Iowa. Her one cousin was kind of scared of her. I guess she thought she would break if she held her.

On *October 23rd* Krista rolled completely over and was really shocked. Then she started rolling from her tummy to her back.

On *November 21st* our girl found her feet and started playing with them. She started sitting alone, too.

Krista had to spend time at babysitter's or with Grandma Heupel in the summer when Mom was out helping in the field. At one babysitter's she got bit. She would never go back there again.

In the fall of 1986 she went with us in the truck to haul bales. She liked watching her Dad load bales onto the truck.

Her first trip to visit Grandma and Grandpa Larsen was at Thanksgiving in 1986.

Krista started drinking from a cup in December. She also started moving a ball and she sat up good by herself. She got her first tooth. She didn't like peas though. She would shake her head and spit them out.

When Krista was 1 ½ years old, we moved from the farm we were at to Elmer's folks' farm three miles north. When I was working on the house, she came up behind me and bit me. I scolded her. Grandma and Grandpa Heupel were upset with me, but I told them she has to learn to not bite people.

One babysitter where she went, the family had three young girls. They took Krista to the Elgin Swimming Pool. They also taught her how to color. They were really good to her. She loved it there.

When Krista was three she ended up in the hospital with a bladder infection. The nurses couldn't find a vein and they kept sticking her. Finally one nurse got the IV in. To this day Krista hasn't forgotten that experience.

I took Krista to Kid's Club at Mott, ND. So she would get out with other kids and meet more kids. She loved it.

Krista loved to go to Grandma and Grandpa Larsen's farm at Epping, ND, to play with her cousins. She loved to blow bubbles with her cousins. The cousins also liked to go outside at the farm and fly kites that Grandma Larsen had bought for them. Some of kites got hung up in the tall trees at the farm.

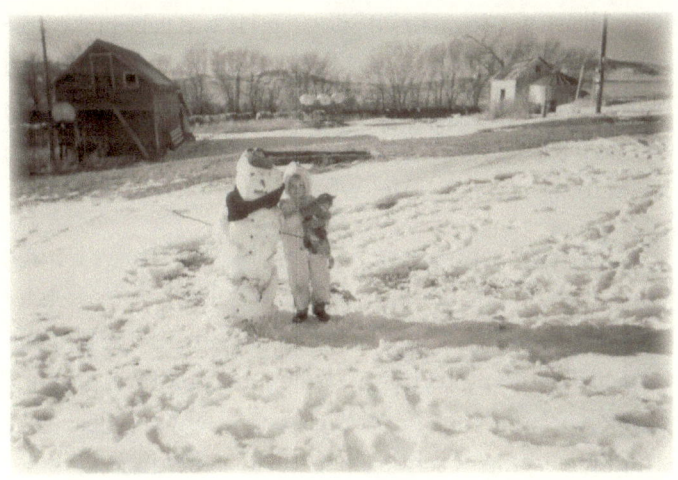

Krista & her snowman & Missy the cat 1989

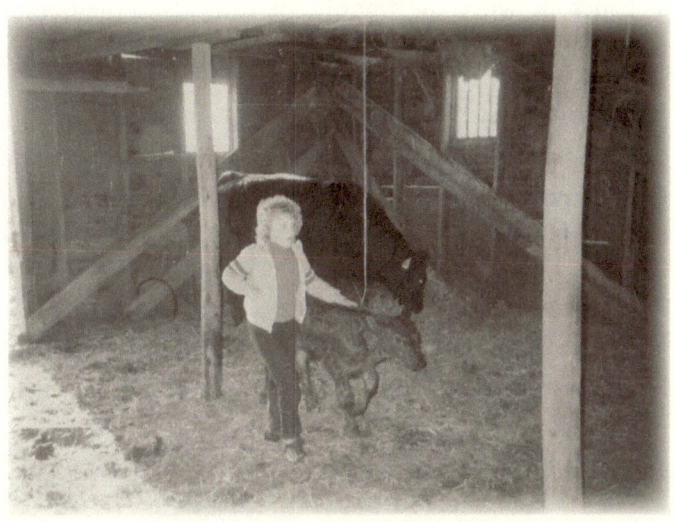

Krista tending a calf 1993

Krista had a pet dog named Snoozer. He was very protective of her. She also had several cats. She loved to watch the baby calves in the springtime. She loved to be outside in the yard swinging in her swing. In the summertime she loved to play in her little swimming pool.

Krista started kindergarten when she was five years old. One day she got scared and she wouldn't go to school the next day. I had to ride the bus with Krista and her Dad had to come to town to pick me up. That was one of the hardest things I ever did in my life was to leave my daughter crying at school, but it had to be done.

When our girl was young she loved to go to the Sesame Street Performances in Bismarck, ND. I also went with as a chaperone when the school took the kids to the Circus in Bismarck.

Krista joined Girl Scouts when she was in first grade. She earned her Gold Award as a senior in High School. She took piano lessons for five years and loved to sing solos in Church. She played flute for Band and sang in the Choir at school.

Krista did well in school. She loved to be read to from little on and she still loves to read. She also did well in math and went to the Math Meets. She got to go to several Spelling Bees at Carson, ND.

Our girl loved to go to Sunday school and be in the Christmas Programs at church. She was very fortunate that she got to stay at the New Leipzig School from grades

K through eight, before she had to go to Elgin for High School, when Elgin and New Leipzig combined.

Krista was in a lot of extra-curricular activities in High School. In her sophomore year she went with the FFA to the National FFA Convention in Louisville, Kentucky. She went to the State FFA Conventions in Fargo, ND all four years of her High School.

She was very active in her High School Youth Group. When she was in tenth grade she joined the Carry the Cross Ministry Puppet Team.

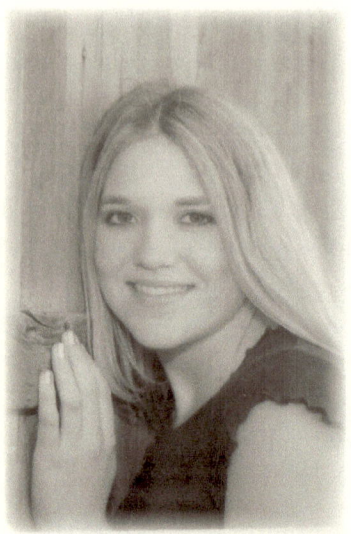

Krista's Graduation Photo

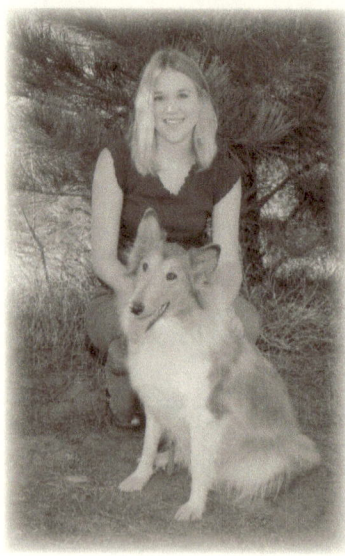

Krista & her Collie dog "Princess" 2004

Krista went on to College at the University of Mary in Bismarck, ND.

Krista's freshmen year of college, during her spring break, she went to Panama City, Florida with the Campus Crusade for Christ Group. She thoroughly enjoyed her trip and would like to go back again someday. That following summer she chaperoned High School Students on a Missions trip to Chicago, Illinois.

Krista graduated on May 3, 2008 with a Major in Social Work and a minor in Sociology from the University of Mary in Bismarck, ND.

All Elmer and I prayed for was to have a healthy baby. We were blessed to have a healthy baby girl and she has grown up to be a healthy young lady who loves the Lord and wants to help people with her Social Work Degree. Krista was employed with the North Dakota Teen Challenge in Mandan, ND.

Krista's parents both grew up on farms. Krista's Dad, Elmer grew up on a farm 3 ½ miles south of New Leipzig, ND. He went to four years of High School in New Leipzig, N.D. After High School Elmer went to two quarters of college at Dickinson State Teacher's College. Then he came back to the farm and worked at various jobs. In January of 1964 Elmer entered the US Army and was discharged in December of 1965. He had a tour of duty in Germany for 18 months. In September of 1966 Elmer started College at NDSU in Fargo, N.D. Elmer graduated from NDSU at the end of the summer session in 1969. He pursued a degree in Ag Economics. Elmer got a job in Beulah, N.D. in September of 1969 at the PCA Office, which is now called Farm Credit Services. Elmer worked there until the end of September in 1970. Then he was transferred to the Watford City Office in October of 1970. He worked there until March of 1972. He bought a farm 6 miles south of New Leipzig, N.D. and started his farming and ranching career.

Diane grew up on a farm 9 miles north of Epping, N.D.. She went to a country school through the eighth grade. She graduated from Williston High School and went on to the UND Williston Center and pursued a degree as a secretary. Diane worked at the Williston High School as secretary to the Principal from 1966 until June of 1974. On weekends during the summer months Diane would go back to the farm and help her parents with haying and harvesting.

Diane moved to the farm 6 miles south of New Leipzig, the beginning of July in 1974. In November of 1987 Elmer and Diane moved to Elmer's parents' farm and are still living on that farm.

Diane never worked off the farm. Diane has worked on the farm with Elmer for the past 38 years.

Diane and Elmer are active members of the Hope Congregational Church in Elgin, N.D. We have served on various jobs in the church. Currently Elmer is serving as Deacon and Diane is a Sunday School Teacher and Sunday School Treasurer. Diane has taught Sunday School since 1979.

Diane has also been a Girl Scout Leader in New Leipzig for 20 years. Diane started helping with Girl Scouts when Krista was in first grade and has continued leading Girl Scouts. This year we currently have 17 Girl Scouts from New Leipzig, Elgin, Carson and Mott.

Elmer and Diane have been married for 38 years and reside on their farm 3 ½ miles south of New Leipzig.

Since I started writing my book Krista got married to Michael Erickson in Bismarck, ND at the New Song Church on June 11, 2010.

Right before Krista and Mike were married Krista was approached about opening a Day Care Center at the New Song Church. Right after Krista and Mike were married, Krista worked for 2 ½ months working on setting up the Daycare. In August of 2010 the Daycare opened. Krista is still the Director of Daycare and her husband is the Facility Manager of the New Song Church.

Krista and Mike feel blessed to be working at the church. They have so many Christian friends.

As the title of my book says Patiently Waiting, it is true we waited patiently for a long time for our lovely daughter. We had many ups and downs along the way, but in the end it was worth it and we were truly blessed by the Lord to have a lovely daughter and now have gained a wonderful son-in-law.

This book would have not been possible without the support of my husband Elmer who has been with me every step of the way in our 38 years of marriage. Thank you Elmer for being with me through all of our ups and downs. It has been a journey that hasn't been easy, but with the Lord and with my faithful husband I have made it through the tough times. I love you and would have never made it without you.

Also thank you to my daughter Krista for helping me proof read my book and for being the lovely daughter and friend that you have been to your Mom. I love you and am happy that you have found such a wonderful husband to share the rest of your life with.

I also want to thank my Mom and Dad Larsen who have since passed away for all the help that they gave to Elmer and I throughout the years. It was much appreciated. I miss you both so much and many times I've wanted to call you up and ask you questions, but can't anymore.

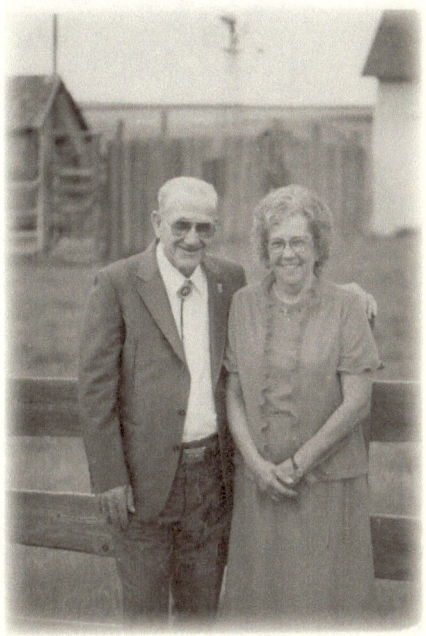

Carl & Ruth Larsen

Thank you also to Mom and Dad Heupel for all the help they have given us over the years also. Dad Heupel has passed away, but Mom Heupel is still with us and we are still fortunate to have her with us.

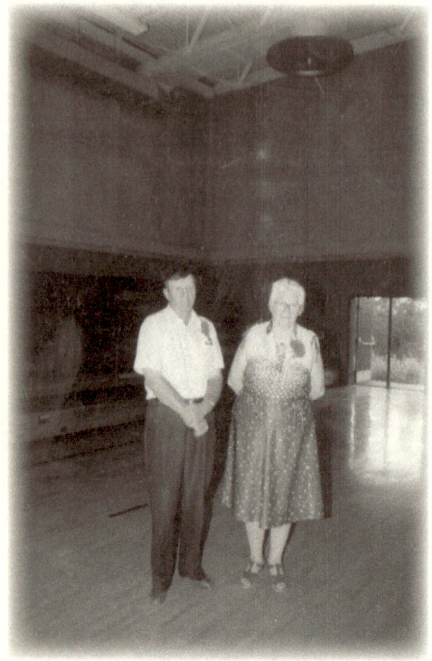

Art & Martha Heupel

To all of my siblings and Elmer's siblings I thank you for all the support you have given us through all that Elmer and I went through.

I am thankful to Hope Congregational Church in Elgin, ND for being there for Elmer and I over the years. We appreciate our Church Family.

Thank you to all of our friends that have given us support throughout the tough times that we went through.